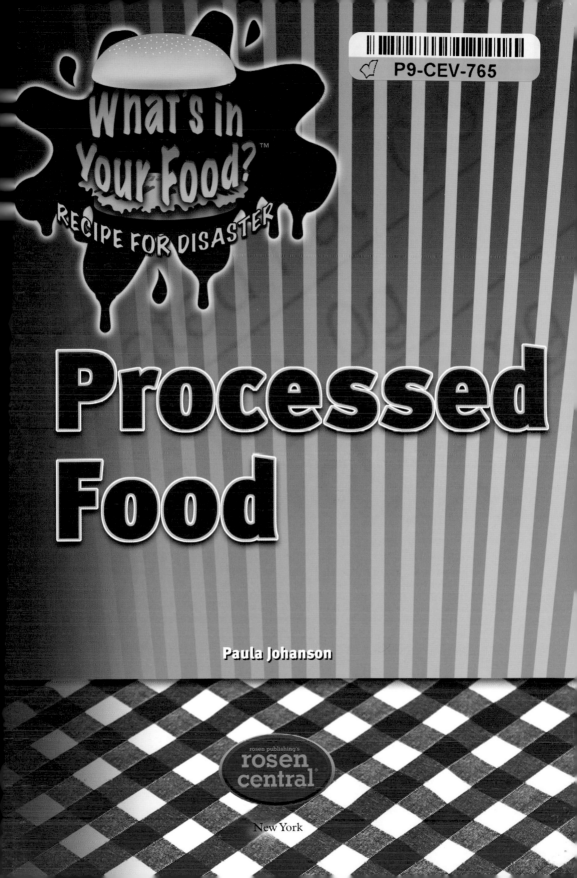

What's in Your Food?™

RECIPE FOR DISASTER

Processed Food

Paula Johanson

rosen publishing's
rosen central

New York

To Sunnyside and DoubleJoy Farms.
For that which we are about to receive, may we be truly thankful.

Published in 2008 by The Rosen Publishing Group, Inc.
29 East 21st Street, New York, NY 10010

Library of Congress Cataloging-in-Publication Data

Johanson, Paula.
Processed food / Paula Johanson.—1st ed.
    p. cm.—(What's in your food? Recipe for disaster)
Includes bibliographical references and index.
ISBN-13: 978-1-4042-1417-0 (library binding: alk. paper)
1. Food adulteration and inspection. I. Title.
TX531.J64 2007
363.19'26—dc22

                                                                    2007028434

Manufactured in China

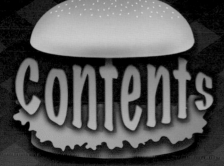

Contents

Introduction

What did you eat yesterday? Did you drink milk or soda? Maybe you made a sandwich or bought a slice of pizza. Did you have salad or canned soup? If you're like most North Americans, more than half of the food you ate in the last few days was processed food.

Since the 1950s, there has been a surprising expansion of a new kind of product for sale: processed food. It is food that has been prepared and packaged in factories, then shipped to stores. Previously, most people cooked their food at home or ate at restaurants. Now, instead of buying dry beans or even a can of cooked beans, you can buy a can of chili con carne ready-made. Processed food usually costs a lot more than the uncooked ingredients. But most North Americans find processed food convenient. Sometimes, that's the only food sold in nearby stores.

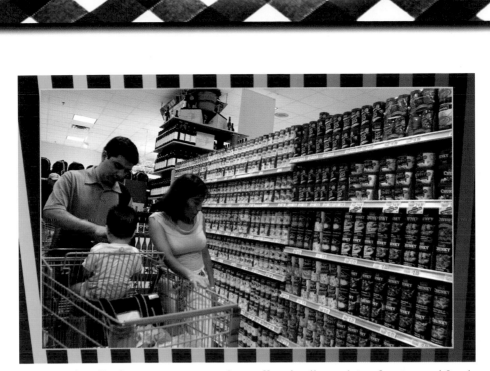

Supermarket displays are set up to show off and sell a variety of processed food. Stores make more money from selling processed food than from whole grains, vegetables, and fruits.

It seems to be modern, efficient, and effective to buy processed food. Why should busy people spend time cooking instead of working or having fun? If you can't hire a cook, at least you can afford to buy food that is already made! But it's becoming popular again for some people to enjoy cooking, barbecuing, or baking for special occasions. Others cook most of the time to take advantage of good-quality ingredients that are affordable.

People do worry about their food, and with good reason. This year, more than 300,000 Americans will go to the hospital because of the food they eat, according to food journalists Alisa Smith and James MacKinnon. A third of Canadians will suffer some kind of food-related illness, usually no worse than diarrhea. But the CDC (Centers for Disease Control and Prevention) is still investigating illnesses caused by processed food in 2006 and 2007, such as peanut butter tainted with *Salmonella* bacteria in a Georgia factory, and lettuce and bags of prewashed spinach contaminated with *E. coli* bacteria. People worry whether children will be affected.

A lot of processed food is marketed for children, just like fashionable clothing and new cars are marketed for adults. Some parents, schools, and young people believe it is wrong to make advertisements aimed at children. Ads promoting cigarettes and alcohol to children are no longer made, but it may be the same kind of exploitation when processed food products are promoted to children.

Over the last sixty years, more and more of the food North Americans eat has become so processed that it's hard to see anything of the original plant or animal. The processed food products have more calories than do fruits and vegetables or grains. That makes it easier for people to eat too many calories. Two-thirds of Americans over the age of twenty are overweight, according to the CDC's National Health and Nutrition Examination Survey, and a third are considered obese. Processed food products also have fewer nutrients, so people may be missing several important vitamins and minerals. The result means bad health for more North Americans each year, from diabetes, cardiovascular problems, and cancer to simply catching colds more frequently.

Chapter One

What Is Processed Food?

Food starts out as plants. These plants may grow wild or grow as crops in farms and greenhouses. People eat the flowers and fruits of plants such as broccoli or strawberries. They eat the leaves, stems, and roots of plants such as lettuce, celery, and carrots. They gather seafood from the ocean, or raise some fish in large nets. The animals that people raise for food eat grass, grains, and other plants, too.

Some food you eat raw, right where it grows. But most food gets washed and cut into pieces. Grains are cracked or ground into flour. When a farm crop is ready to harvest, there's more than all the people nearby can eat right away, so it has to be kept from spoiling. People preserve food by freezing, drying, or sealing it in airtight packages such as cans, jars, or plastic containers. Some food gets cooked to soften it and kill germs. People mix various foods together, making bread or casseroles or sauces.

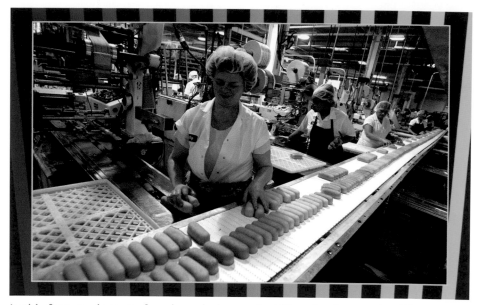

In this factory, dozens of workers during each shift make thousands of little cakes every day, all exactly alike. They use different ingredients than those found in homemade cake recipes.

All that washing, cutting, preserving, cooking, and mixing are processes to prepare food for eating. You can process food in your own home. If you grow tomatoes that ripen all at once, then you might have to process them into spaghetti sauce.

When food is processed for sale, more than one meal is made. Each batch of processed food may have hundreds or thousands of servings. Each serving is like all the others. The processing is done in a factory with cooking pots the size of bathtubs and hot tubs. The ovens and freezers can be as large as garages. Some factories have conveyor belts moving ingredients from one machine to another.

Processed food is sold in many forms. It comes as baked goods and pasta made from refined white flour. There are also cans of cooked and seasoned vegetables and fruits, meat, and fish products. Ready-to-eat frozen or canned foods, snack foods, cookies, and sugary breakfast cereals are convenient. There are packages for making dinners by adding meat or other proteins to sauce mixes.

Supermarket Displays

When you enter a supermarket or large grocery store, there's a bewildering variety of food on display. Boxes, bags, cans, and bottles of processed food dominate the center aisles. You have to walk past them to find fresh fruits and vegetables, or go to the back of the super-market to find the baked goods and dairy products. That's on purpose. When you come to the store to buy milk, bread, and fruit, you end up seeing soft drinks, snacks, and ready-made dinners first.

The stores and the food wholesalers make the most profit from selling processed food. What started out as a corncob or a potato has become a "value-added product." We can understand that a pair of blue jeans costs more than a pile of cotton fluff just picked. The cotton has been washed, carded, spun, dyed, woven, and sewn into a garment. Someone added value to the product. But most processed food is not only washed, cut, and preserved. Highly processed foods have many nutrients removed and many ingredients added that

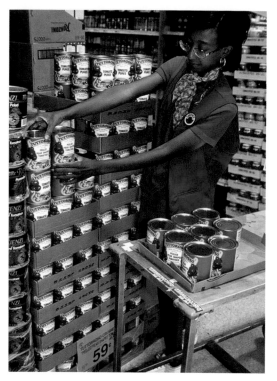

Here, a worker stacks cans of Italian tomatoes. The canning process can preserve food from far away and allow food to be transported anywhere. But you may be surprised at what exotic or ordinary food is available locally grown and fresh!

you wouldn't use at home. It's as if that cotton was mixed with other fibers to make blue jeans that looked good but didn't last. The foods that bring the most profit to the stores, and the wholesalers, are not the foods that are cheap and most nutritious to eat.

It seems as though most North Americans have a lot of food choices available. But most of them don't eat a varied diet. "Unbelievable as it may seem," said nutritionist Marion Nestle in her book *What to Eat*, "one-third of all vegetables consumed in the United States come from just three sources: French fries, potato chips, and iceberg lettuce." Two of those sources are processed food made from potatoes deep-fried in fat. Add canned tomato products, and that makes half of all vegetables Americans eat.

Anonymous Food

When you catch a fish, you know where it was swimming. But where did all the fish come from that were made into thousands of frozen fish sticks? Processed food is more likely to contain environmental contaminants than unprocessed meat, fish, or produce in general because the ingredients are more anonymous. It's hard to tell just which fish in a big batch of canned fish product was the one with the mercury taint.

Manufacturers put batch numbers on bags, boxes, and cans, along with a sell-by date. Sometimes, there are notices on television, radio, in newspapers, and in stores to recall a batch of processed food because of an environmental or microbial contaminant.

Contamination

The factories where food is processed can have the same problems as any factory. Dust and bugs may blow in through air vents. Rats and mice may bring germs that make people sick. Machinery may break down and let dirty grease or bolts fall into the food. There are very strict government regulations for worker safety and food safety in factories. But these regulations acknowledge that a few insects, rodent hairs, and droppings just might end up in a batch of hot dogs or cans of food. If that bothers you, then remember that foods sold as kosher (suitable for

Myths & Facts

Myth: Food is food—it doesn't matter whether you eat one thing or another.

Fact: All food is not alike. Some processed foods such as candy are made of only sugar and have no proteins, fats, vitamins, minerals, or fiber to help you be healthy.

Myth: I eat what I like.

Fact: You eat what you've got. If all you have to eat is canned goods or bags of snacks, then you won't know whether you like home-cooked food and fresh vegetables. Choose healthy foods and you'll find you will like many kinds of food.

Myth: I can't afford to eat better food.

Fact: Potato chips cost eight to ten times as much as fresh potatoes. Processed foods have more calories but less nutrition than fresh fruits, vegetables, and whole grains. You are buying good health when you buy whole, fresh foods.

Myth: Only crazy people panic about perfectly good processed food.

Fact: Doctors, scientists, businesspeople, and families are all looking for food that is nutritious, tasty, and affordable.

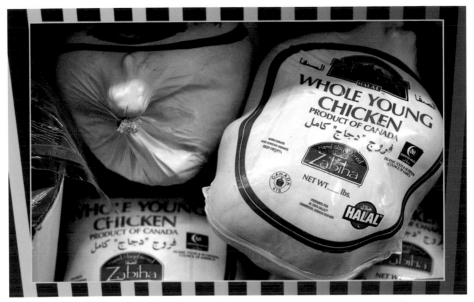

We cook meat not only to make the proteins more digestible but also to kill germs. Some religious groups have strict food rules for cleanliness and humane butchering of animals.

Jewish diets) or halal (suitable for Muslim diets) have stricter rules for cleanliness that are set by the factories themselves and by religious groups.

Processed food can be contaminated with bacteria from manure. *Escherichia coli* is a bacterium that lives in animal and human bowels. Usually it's harmless. But one variety, *E. coli* 0157:H7, is resistant to antibiotics and can cause death. It's commonly found in feedlot cattle being slaughtered for processed meat products. The worry is not only for anyone eating processed meat products that haven't been cooked enough to kill the microbes. It's also a particular concern for people who are young, elderly, and ill, and those who are

13

taking antibiotics. They are more susceptible to harm from the microbes.

When Food Goes Bad

Other processed food contamination concerns are for microbes such as botulism. Botulism and other microbes that make food spoil are common in dirt and dust, and they are blown in the wind. That's part of why we cook food—to kill germs.

We seal cans or jars to keep the germs in dirt and air out of clean food. But if the cans or jars weren't sealed tight or not cooked long enough, microbes can grow and spoil the food. Sometimes, you can tell without opening the jar because you can see a clump of mold, or perhaps juice that should be clear is cloudy. If a can is bulging, dented, or bent, do not use it. Damaged cans often get leaks and make food spoil.

If a can of peaches goes bad, you can usually smell or taste it and wouldn't eat more than a lick. But if a can or jar of food containing a lot of spices and garlic spoils, it's harder to tell. This is one reason why it's a good idea to eat fresh fruits and vegetables and meats. You always can add seasoning while cooking. Processed foods are seasoned with a lot of salt and other cheap spices. If you ever help someone who is preserving fruit or jam in sterilized Mason jars, then you'll see how the instructions must be followed exactly in order to kill all germs and seal the jars tightly for food safety.

Chapter Two

How Is It Made?

Where does your food come from? Does it come from your garden? Do you go to a nearby farm to get vegetables and fruits? Many North Americans, even farmers, get most of their food from a store, and most of that food was not grown nearby. It was carried on trucks, trains, and airplanes for hundreds of miles or across the country. Your dinner's footprint is larger than the field where the plants grew because of this shipping. The ecological impact usually stretches 1,500 to 3,000 miles (2,414 to 4,828 kilometers) from farm to plate, according to the Leopold Center for Sustainable Agriculture in Ames, Iowa.

Processed food is shipped several times: from the farm to the slaughterhouse or warehouse and to the factory, and then from the factory to another warehouse and eventually to the store. That uses a lot of fuel for transportation. If you drive a car to

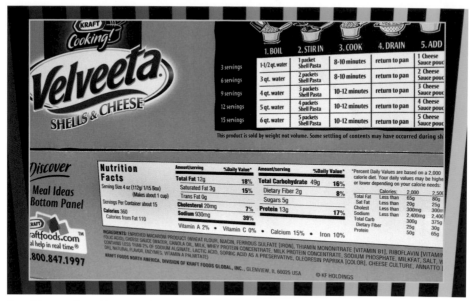

Read ingredient lists on the nutrition label when you shop for processed food. There's more of the first item, and less of each item as you read along the list. See if preservatives, fake color, salt, and sugar have been added.

the store, then that's one more use of fuel, but it's the easiest one to avoid. For half the price of a tank of gas, you can get a little folding cart or a wagon that will last for years. Walking to the store is healthy exercise. You should plan ahead for trips to the store so that you can save on gas.

How Much Processing

Some food doesn't get processed very much. You can grow a head of lettuce, wash it, and cut it up for salad. Or you can buy prewashed romaine lettuce hearts, or a precut salad with little bags of dressing and croutons.

These foods are at risk for contamination with *E. coli* and other germs. Some frozen vegetables are just washed, cut up, and flash-frozen. These keep more nutrients than if the same vegetables were kept in a cooler for many months.

Other processed food has been cooked with many ingredients added to change the color, flavor, texture, and appearance. "If you want healthier frozen foods," said nutritionist Marion Nestle, "look for packages with shorter ingredients lists."

You can bake a cake at home with as few as six ingredients. But a commercially made cake such as a Twinkie has thirty-nine ingredients or more. Some of these keep the cake from spoiling inside its wrapper. Other ingredients replace the butter and cream in a homemade cream cake with harmful trans fats and slippery cooked cotton cellulose.

Most processed foods have corn products or soy products added because American farms grow a lot of corn and soybeans. Very little corn and soy is used whole. Most is cooked or ground, and split into oil, syrup, protein, starch, and other products that are mixed into almost every kind and brand of processed food.

Standardized Ingredients

When people cook at home, they use a variety of recipes. Maybe your family has a favorite way to make bread. Your friend may cook omelets differently every time, using peppers or asparagus. The best clam chowder is made in seaside towns where clams are gathered. Some families make meals that are part of their heritage, using special ingredients and methods. This diversity makes for interesting meals as well as a mix of nutrients.

Processed food uses standard recipes. A packaged macaroni-and-cheese dinner sold in Seattle is sold in Miami, too. The company that owns the factory uses a recipe for large quantities of ingredients. It makes the exact same packaged dinner over and over again. When a company develops a new recipe, it's not like your friend cooking an omelet with asparagus in April. New processed food recipes are designed like new clothes marketed by fashion designers. The company wants a new product it can sell for more money.

When manufacturers treat food as if it was the new style of jacket everyone is wearing, people lose some of their cultural and local diversity. When manufacturers treat food like a stack of bricks that are all the same, consumers should insist that at least the food should be nutritious, but they don't. In Great Britain and Finland, laws have been passed to limit the amount of salt added to processed food. In Europe, labels must show if a processed food contains genetically modified organisms.

Factory Farming Methods

A few animals on small farms are raised organically, without chemicals except medicine if they have an injury. The cows and sheep eat grass and hay, and the chickens and pigs eat grains and weeds, their natural foods. The animals have a field to graze and water to drink. There's usually a shed or barn for shelter or shade.

But most chickens that are raised for meat in super-markets and processed food live in stacked wire cages for all their lives. They don't walk around scratching for weeds and bugs to eat, so their meat and eggs are less tasty and nutritious.

Most pigs that are raised for supermarkets and processed food live in wire cages, too, stacked three or four high in some barns. If they're able to walk around, then it's in a pen so crowded with other pigs that their sharp teeth must be broken off and their tails cut short so that they don't bite each other.

The life of a young steer grazing on a ranch is similar to the life of wild bison roaming the prairie. But the last five months of a steer's life are spent on a feedlot. There, steers are fenced into small yards and are fed

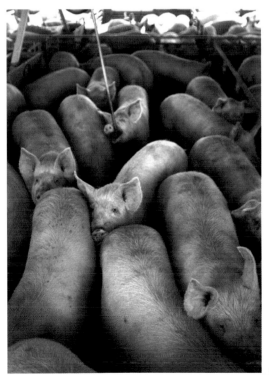

The pig in the middle is drinking from a hose. Pigs raised for processed food live short, crowded, unhappy lives.

19

corn. Bovine stomachs aren't adapted to corn, so they're given antibiotics to reduce the stomach and liver problems it causes. The feed is also mixed with beef fat and beef blood.

Some feedlots and factory farms mix ground-up animal bits and the litter from chicken barns into animal feed. The law was changed in 1997 so that animals are no longer fed meat from the same kind of animal, but cattle are fed chicken and pig meal, and pigs and chicken are fed bovine meal. The idea was to reduce the risk of mad cow disease spreading among cattle.

In the feedlots and barns of stacked cages, manure piles up underfoot. It gets hosed away as runoff. The runoff is toxic with so much nitrogen, phosphorus, antibiotics, and hormones that it can't be used as fertilizer. The runoff from factory farms and corn farming runs down the Mississippi River into the Gulf of Mexico. There, so much algae feeds on the nitrogen that for 8,000 square miles (20,720 square kilometers) of ocean, there's no oxygen for anything else to live.

Slaughterhouses

The meat in supermarkets and processed meat comes from large slaughterhouses, where every day hundreds of animals are butchered. Instead of washing manure and dirt off the carcass with a simple hose, workers use a pressure washer that forces tiny bits of manure into the meat. The federal meat inspectors order workers to cut any visible tumors off a carcass. Most inspectors do not have time to look all over both sides of a large carcass.

Some meat packers use hydrolyzed pork and beef proteins, extracted from old animals or from skin and bone, to bulk up chicken. When mixed with water and injected into a chicken carcass, the meat swells. The meat packer is able to sell water at the same price-per-pound as chicken. The process is only illegal if the meat is incorrectly labeled. The swollen chicken meat is marketed to caterers, pubs, clubs, wholesalers, and ethnic restaurants, and it is used by manufacturers for processed meat products.

Catching Fish

Most fish in processed food is not caught on a hook and line. Wild fish are usually caught in big nets that kill many kinds of fish. The unwanted ones are thrown back. Some nets are dragged across the sea bottom, breaking the coral where tiny fish live. It gets harder each year to find the kinds of fish that many people like to eat.

Raising fish in fish farms is not the best alternative. Farmed salmon just doesn't taste as good. The nets are often small and allow Atlantic salmon to escape into Pacific waters. Sea lice thrive on the small fish and spread to nearby wild salmon.

But there is good news about tuna. All canned tuna now carries the "dolphin-friendly" symbol to show that no dolphins were killed when the tuna was caught.

21

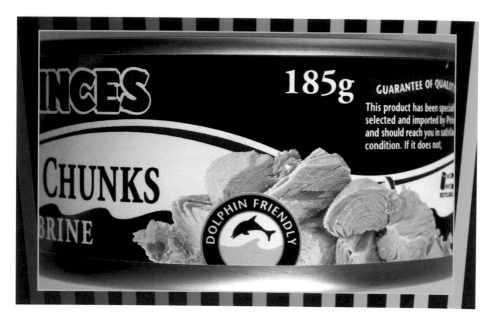

Even big corporations respond to laws and public opinion. Now, all canned tuna is caught without drowning dolphins, as this dolphin-friendly label attests.

Public outrage about dolphins drowning in nets caused the fish canning industry to change its methods.

Packaging

Most processed food is packaged in plastic or is sealed in cans. This covering seals in the food and keeps out air and germs so that the food doesn't go bad. Plastic is usually stiff and brittle unless certain petrochemicals are added to it, like bisphenol A or phthalates. These petrochemicals make plastic flexible. Tin cans may have a lining to prevent the food from touching the metal. Even though the container is called "food grade," some chemicals soak into the food. People who eat very little processed food can taste a "plasticky," chemical taste on some foods in plastic packages, sandwich bags, or plastic wrap.

Phthalates have an effect like hormones on human and animal bodies. A tiny amount of phthalate in the daily food of millions of people adds up over time, to increase cancer rates and miscarriages, and lower men's sperm counts. Moreover, some scientists interviewed in 2007 for the Canadian newspaper the *Globe and Mail* described bisphenol A as one of "the scariest manufactured substances in use, an eerie modern version of the vaunted lead [water] pipes by which the ancient Romans were unknowingly poisoned."

Never microwave food in a plastic container or cling wrap. This softens some of the chemicals in the plastic and pushes them into the food.

The packaging itself makes garbage. If you peel potatoes for dinner, then the potato peels compost into dirt in a couple of weeks. But if you buy a bag of frozen potato product, then the plastic bag will sit in a garbage dump for years without rotting—and groundwater soaking through that dump will be tainted with plastic and phthalates or bisphenol A.

Chapter Three

What Difference Does It Make?

What difference does it make if many people eat mostly processed food? Well, what people put into their bodies affects their health gradually. When many people eat mostly processed food for years, their health is compromised.

Nutrition

Processed food is usually a reliable source of fuel for quick energy from sugar, simple carbohydrates, and fat. But food should have more than fuel to give you energy. Food should include nutrients such as proteins and fats, which are used for the building blocks that make up your skin, muscles, organs, and bones. Your body uses vitamins and minerals for various functions inside your cells. The nutrients your body uses are naturally present in plants and animals. When you eat a variety of natural and fresh foods, you get all the vitamins, minerals, fats, and proteins your body needs. Sometimes, a doctor will prescribe a particular diet or vitamin pills for pregnant women or people who have been ill so that they can get all of their necessary nutrients.

The vitamins in cheap pills are usually by-products of food processing. Vitamin B pills are made from the hulls of grain, polished off before the kernel of grain is ground into flour. Eat brown rice and whole-wheat flour instead of cheating yourself out of healthy vitamins and fiber!

If you eat only processed food that's missing vitamins and minerals, then your health will suffer. You could get scurvy from a lack of vitamin C; scurvy makes teeth fall out and small cuts that won't heal. A lack of vitamin B causes beriberi and pellagra. Rickets, a condition of weak bones, is caused by a lack of vitamin D. Children who don't eat enough protein develop kwashiorkor. Any of these illnesses makes it harder for young people to grow strong or get well from injuries and colds. Adults suffer even more illness and disabilities.

Additives

Processed food has additives such as preservatives, texture changers, food dyes, and monosodium glutamate (MSG). Gracelyn Guyol, a scholar of brain health, said if you took all the additives out of one serving of processed food, then the additives would make a lump as big as a pill of medicine. Food additives have effects just like medicines do. Nitrates and nitrites keep deli meats from spoiling and increase the risk of cancer.

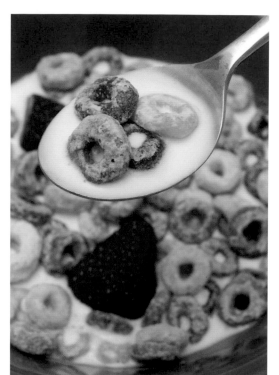

What's in your breakfast bowl? This cereal has a candy bar's worth of sugar. Food additives give color and texture, but even one serving affects some people badly.

Other additives affect the brain and nervous system, increasing the risk of seizures, migraine headaches, and depression.

If you eat one bowl of sugary cereal with colored marshmallows, then you might not notice any effect unless you have an allergy to corn. But if a child eats the same bowl of cereal and has a reaction to the red food dye in that cereal, then the child might be hyperactive that day and find it hard to behave well at school.

Bowel Health

The fiber in food has an effect on your intestines and lower bowel. Food that has a lot of soluble fiber, like cooked oatmeal, brings more water with it into your lower bowel. Food that has a lot of insoluble fiber, like celery, keeps its texture. Both kinds of fiber are necessary for your intestines and keep them working well.

People who eat only processed food or mushy foods may find that their digestion gets slower. Their bowels don't move regularly. A person who eats balanced meals should also be going to the bathroom regularly. People who get constipated are much more likely to have bowel problems. Hemorrhoids or diverticulosis start as small, painful problems and can end up needing surgery. Some research suggests that a lack of fiber can cause colon cancer. It is recommended that you eat twenty-five to thirty grams of fiber per day.

If you're not used to eating fresh fruits and vegetables, then start with one serving at a time, gradually replacing servings of processed foods. Your bowel will get used to the fiber and become regular. A healthy bowel absorbs nutrients better from your food. Sometimes, even food allergies will get partly better. Ask your doctor.

The Effect of Diet on Teeth

Your parents or dentist may have told you that if you eat candy without brushing your teeth afterward, then you are likely to get cavities. The sugar clings to your teeth, and the microbes that normally live on and between your teeth eat the sugar. These microbes live on the complex carbohydrates in fruits, vegetables, and grains, but the simple carbohydrate in refined sugar is a powerful energy source. The microbes eat it, multiply, and their acid wastes make your teeth decay. Candy, soda, cake, and even sticky dried fruit all encourage tooth decay.

27

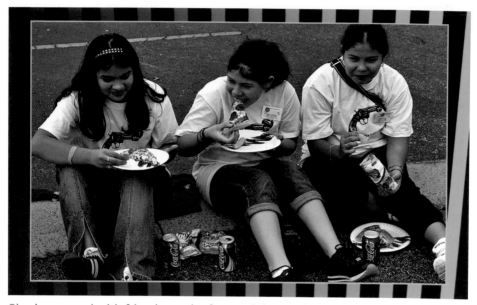

Sharing a meal with friends can be fun, and the meal doesn't have to be bad for your body. Instead of consuming fast-food pizza and soft drinks, go for nutritious food and fruit juice. Start such good habits now.

Do you have cavities? Your ancestors from long ago almost never had tooth decay. When they ate sweet fruit, the fiber in the fruit rubbed their teeth much cleaner than when you eat candy. Medical records around the world show that during the last 500 years, whenever refined sugar became available in a nation, the number of people with tooth decay increased dramatically.

Eating processed foods has other effects. People from long ago chewed on whole grains instead of bread made from refined flour. They ate vegetables and fruits, mostly raw, instead of pies and potato chips. When they ate meat, it was tough and chewy because the animal ran around looking for food instead of living in a tiny cage and eating grain. The hard work of chewing made jaw muscles strong. It even made jaws grow a little bigger than they do today. But now people eat mostly soft food all through childhood. Dentists often have to pull out a person's wisdom teeth because there isn't enough room for them in the jaw.

These wisdom teeth are often softer than normal if a person hasn't been eating enough calcium and other minerals to strengthen the teeth. Some babies' teeth decay easily because their mothers didn't eat enough calcium and other minerals when they were pregnant.

Cardiovascular Health

The saturated fats and trans fats in processed food cause cholesterol and triglycerides to accumulate in your blood. This leads to plaque, which can block blood vessels anywhere in your body. Blocked vessels in your organs or limbs can affect your health for years and can result in a fatal heart attack or stroke. Cardiovascular problems are rare when people eat mostly fresh and unprocessed food. However, cardio-vascular disease is becoming increasingly common in North America, even among young adults.

Autoimmune System Illnesses

People who are vulnerable to arthritis are more likely to get it when they eat processed foods that have a lot of corn, wheat, and milk proteins added. These allergens

29

and other food additives can also cause problems for people with autism, epilepsy, migraines, and depression. The increase in these and other autoimmune system illnesses over the last sixty years is due in part to the interaction between vulnerable genes and environmental triggers, which may cause chronic inflammation.

Food Allergies

Allergies of all kinds have been increasing over the last forty years in North America. One cause has been the use of corn, wheat, milk, and soy in most kinds of processed food. Early childhood exposure to these foods can cause food allergies, and multiple exposures can increase food sensitivity. You may not even know that you have a food allergy, if you think all allergies make people swell up and stop breathing. Even minor food allergies can contribute to rashes, behavior problems, and neurological symptoms.

Is Fat All Bad?

It can be easy to eat more fat than your body needs if you eat a lot of processed food with fat added. But eating healthy food doesn't mean eating no fat. Fat and oil in your food tastes good for a reason. Fat plays a vital role in the health of your body. You must include healthy fats in your diet. Your early ancestors ate a wide variety of plants, fish, and animals. Being human means that our bodies need the vitamins and minerals

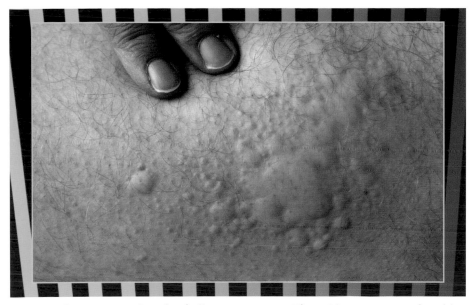

Pay attention to even minor food allergy symptoms. These hives are uncomfortable. So are rashes, behavior problems, and headaches. Choosing food carefully can even save a life.

in many kinds of fats. As Gracelyn Guyol pointed out, the brain is 60 percent fat by weight. Our brains, nerves, cell membranes, and hormones need fat, especially the kinds called fatty omega-3, 6, and 9 acids.

Also, our early ancestors needed every calorie they could get, and fat has nine calories per gram—twice as much as are in carbohydrates or proteins. It's hard to eat too much fat if you get it by cracking walnuts, picking a ripe avocado, or catching a fish. It's even hard to eat too much animal fat if you get it by catching a pheasant or working with other hunters to catch a deer.

Chapter Four

Making Healthy Choices

Every day, you make food choices that can influence your health. Eating a variety of fresh foods makes your body strong so that you're less likely to suffer illness. People who eat well are much less likely to have problems with their lungs, heart, and other organs. Even if someone gets hurt in an accident or gets cancer, eating well helps. But when millions of people choose to eat mostly processed foods, researchers see an increase in bad health. Greater numbers of people are obese and have problems with their bowels, livers, heart, and circulation systems. These health problems aren't accidents. People can choose to have fewer health problems, just like they can choose to cross a street safely.

Breakfast Alternatives

Is your typical breakfast toasted white bread with lots of hard margarine and jelly, a bowl of sugary cereal, and a glass of artificial orange juice? Then you can do a lot better! Try making oatmeal from rolled oats or other whole grains. Cook up a pot for everyone in your family, or pour half a cup of boiling water on a half cup of rolled oats in your bowl. Whole grains have more nutrients and fiber, which is better for your bowels. You can sweeten oatmeal with raisins or other dried or fresh fruit. Or sprinkle in some cinnamon. Adding one spoonful of sugar is better than the five or six in a bowl of commercial cereal.

If you really like toast and jelly, then you can toast bread made from whole grains. Use a little butter or none, instead of hard margarine. Instead of buying jelly,

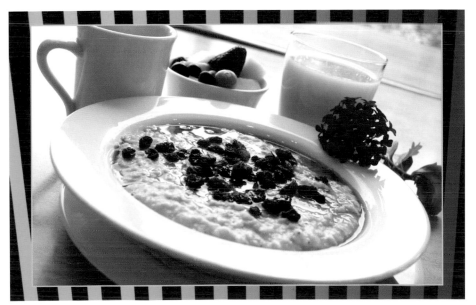

Breakfast with oatmeal, fruit, juice, and milk tastes great. It gives you lasting energy, instead of the short jolt of a cola and frosted boxed cereal, and it costs less!

mash fresh fruit or make sauce from apples and other fruits. You might even try peanut butter or almond butter. As for artificial fruit drinks mixed from powders, fresh-squeezed fruit juice has the same number of calories but also has fiber and a variety of nutrients.

Snack Alternatives

If you're looking for a sweet snack, try fruit or carrots in place of candy. If you like crisp and crackly snacks, try making popcorn. When you're craving salty snacks, be willing to try spicy flavors instead of just salt and fat. Homemade salsa has plenty of flavor. Dried fruit makes a great snack.

Remember when you reach for a snack, you might be thirsty instead of hungry. Drinking five to eight glasses of water each day is good for your body.

Sugar Alternatives

All sweets are not alike to your body. Even though most sugars and carbohydrates have the same number of calories per teaspoon, their effects can be very different. The calories in bread take a while for your body to digest and turn into sugar. But the sugar in corn syrup goes from your digestive system into your blood quickly, and so your pancreas has to make a lot of insulin right away. That will make you feel hungry in about an hour.

Drinking soda is not a good idea. Most sweet, carbonated drinks have five to ten teaspoonfuls of sugar in a single twelve-ounce can. A homemade glass of iced tea usually has only one spoonful! Try fruit juice. It has about as many calories as a can of soda, but it doesn't make your pancreas produce insulin as fast as the corn sugar in soda. Plus, it has vitamins. It's even better for you to eat an apple or pear, and then drink water.

Meat Alternatives

Some people believe that it's healthier to be vegetarian. Others believe that eating meat from healthy animals can be part of a nutritious diet. Meat from animals raised on small farms and organic farms is better for you than meat from animals that were raised in crowded conditions on factory farms. There is less contamination from antibiotics and hormones. Animals are more humanely butchered at a small meat packer, and their meat is inspected more thoroughly, too, than meat sold in supermarkets.

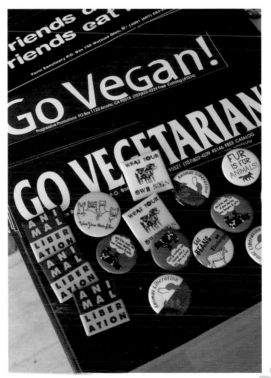

Meat is not necessary for health. Vegetarian food can have all the nutrition you need. There are plenty of vegetarian recipes you can enjoy and vegetarian and vegan diet books at libraries.

Instead of cheap hot dogs, choose locally made high-quality sausages—and make your own hamburger patties instead of buying pre-shaped frozen patties. An even better option is consuming a cut of meat that hasn't been ground up. These choices cost more because you are eating better-quality meat.

Meal Alternatives

If you like the convenience of prepackaged meals, then make meals from scratch and put them in the refrigerator and freezer. You can also package pasta or rice and sauce ingredients, ready to cook. In one afternoon or evening, you can get several meals ready.

You can use or adapt recipes from your own family or culture to make tasty meals with good meat, vegetarian ingredients, or a combination of meat and vegetable proteins. There are lots of cookbooks at the library. Start a cooking group at a local community center, with a nutritionist to give you advice.

Choosing Some Processed Foods

Of course, most people choose to eat processed food sometimes. But it should be a choice and not the only food in the house or the nearest store. If your grandparents want to give you a chocolate bar, or your friend wants to share a bag of potato chips, that's because they want to share a treat. Unless you have a food allergy or are diabetic, one treat like that every

10 Great Questions to Ask

1. What can I eat to improve my health?

2. Is there any food you want me to avoid completely?

3. If one of my relatives is a diabetic, does that mean I'm going to be one, too?

4. Can you give me anything to read about nutrition?

5. How can my diet help me do better at sports?

6. How can my diet help me do well at learning?

7. How can my diet help me if I am pregnant?

8. Where can I get recipes for the food you want me to eat?

9. Is there a local group from which I can learn recipes and how to cook?

10. What if I want to eat well, but a lot of foods just seem yucky or make my stomach hurt?

Cooking is an important part of family life for many people. You can prepare traditional recipes with your family, as well as embrace new foods.

now and then won't cause a big problem.

There are other treats you can share with them. Maybe your grandparents would enjoy showing you how to eat a mango or prickly pear or strawberries, just like they did as children. Maybe you and your friend might make a homemade pizza with whole-wheat crust and fresh toppings—it'll have a lot less salt, sugar, and preservatives than takeout pizza. Your choice to eat more healthy whole foods and less processed foods is something that you, your family, and your friends can enjoy together.

Glossary

allergens Substances, usually proteins, which cause an allergic response such as hives, swelling, stomachaches, hyperactivity, rashes, or breathing problems.

beriberi A disease caused by the lack of thiamine (vitamin B_1) and characterized by inflammation of nerves, heart disease, and swelling of the body's organs.

calories The energy your body gets from food. For instance, carbohydrates and proteins have 4.5 calories per gram, and fat has 9 calories per gram.

chronic Always present, as in a long-lasting disease or condition.

diversity The differences between one similar thing and another. Diversity in genes makes plants and animals able to survive in a variety of conditions.

diverticulosis Bulging, sore places in the colon, where wastes can cause inflammation.

Escherichia coli (E. coli) A bacterium that lives in human and animal intestines. Usually, an *E. coli* infection causes mild diarrhea or no symptoms at all in healthy adults.

fiber Bulky cells in plant and animal tissue that can absorb water or give tough texture to food.

footprint The amount of land it took to grow the plants, and the plants which fed the animals, which became your food.

halal Meeting the diet restrictions for Muslims.

hemorrhoids Sores on the rectum.

hydrolyze To break down into components, as in hydrolyzed protein that has been broken down into amino acids. Hydrolyzed protein often is used to improve food flavor and contains MSG.

kosher Meeting the diet restrictions for Jews.

kwashiorkor An often fatal illness caused by not enough protein in the diet.

monosodium glutamate (MSG) A food additive that causes food allergies and neurological symptoms; it is used in processed foods and as a spice in Asian cooking.

pellagra A disease that occurs when someone does not get enough niacin (a B complex vitamin) in the diet and, as a result, suffers from skin sores, diarrhea, and confusion.

phthalates Chemicals used to soften plastic; they have hormone-like effects on human and animal bodies.

rickets A disease caused by the lack of calcium and phosphorus due to getting little sunlight or vitamin D; it is characterized by soft bones.

Salmonella A bacteria that can grow in food at room temperature; it causes vomiting and severe diarrhea.

Center for Food Safety and Applied Nutrition
U.S. Food and Drug Administration (FDA)
5600 Fishers Lane
Rockville, MD 20857
(888) 463-6332
Web site: http://www.foodsafety.gov
This organization is the FDA's gateway to food safety information for consumers and industry. Articles on food safety and applied nutrition are available at its Web site. Links to news, safety alerts, where to report illnesses and product complaints, and consumer advice are also accessible.

MyPyramid.gov and *USDA Dietary Guidelines (2005)*
U.S. Department of Agriculture (USDA)
USDA Center for Nutrition Policy and Promotion
3101 Park Center Drive, Room 1034
Alexandria, VA 22302-1594
(888) 779-7264
Web site: http://www.mypyramid.gov
This USDA Web site offers users a personal eating plan with healthy food choices and food amounts that are appropriate for individuals. MyPyramid Tracker helps people assess their food choices and physical activity routines.

National Eating Disorders Association (NEDA)
603 Stewart Street, Suite 803
Seattle, WA 98101
(800) 931-2237
Web site: http://www.edap.org
NEDA is the largest nonprofit organization that works
    to prevent eating disorders and help people who are
    suffering from them.

Public Health Agency of Canada
130 Colonnade Road
A. L. 6501H
Ottawa, ON K1A 0K9
Canada
Web site: http://www.hc-sc.gc.ca/index_e.html
The Web site of the organization offers food and
    nutrition advice, Canada's Food Guide, and infor-
    mation about food advisories, warnings, recalls,
    labeling, and safety.

Web Sites

Due to the changing nature of Internet links, Rosen
Publishing has developed an online list of Web sites
related to the subject of this book. This site is updated
regularly. Please use this link to access the list:

http://www.rosenlinks.com/wyf/prfo

For Further Reading

Elgin, Tershia. *What Should I Eat? A Complete Guide to the New Food Pyramid.* New York, NY: Ballantine, 2005.

Ettlinger, Steve. *Twinkie, Deconstructed: My Journey to Discover How the Ingredients Found in Processed Foods Are Grown, Mined (Yes, Mined), and Manipulated into What America Eats.* New York, NY: Hudson Street Press, 2007.

Harmon, Daniel E. *Obesity* (Coping in a Changing World). New York, NY: Rosen Publishing, 2007.

Jamieson, Alex. *The Great American Detox Diet: 8 Weeks to Weight Loss and Well-Being.* New York, NY: Rodale Books, 2005.

Nestle, Marion. *What to Eat.* New York, NY: North Point Press, 2006.

Pawlick, Thomas F. *The End of Food: How the Food Industry Is Destroying Our Food Supply—and What You Can Do About It.* Vancouver, Canada: Greystone Books, 2006.

Salmon, Margaret B. *Food Facts for Teenagers: A Guide to Good Nutrition for Teens and Preteens.* 2nd ed. Springfield, IL: Charles C. Thomas, 2002.

Schlosser, Eric, and Charles Wilson. *Chew on This: Everything You Don't Want to Know About Fast Food.* New York, NY: Houghton Mifflin, 2006.

Schlosser, Eric. *Fast Food Nation.* Boston, MA:
    Houghton Mifflin Company, 2001.
USDA Dietary Guidelines 2005. January 12, 2005.
    Retrieved June 5, 2007 (http://www.health.gov/
    dietaryguidelines/dga2005/document/html/
    executivesummary.htm).
Williams, Kara. *Frequently Asked Questions About
    MyPyramid: Eating Right* (FAQ: Teen Life). New York,
    NY: Rosen Publishing, 2007.

Bibliography

Curtis, Polly. "Cutting Salt 'Reduces Risk of Premature Death.'" *Guardian Unlimited*. Friday, April 20, 2007. Retrieved May 2, 2007 (http://www.guardian.co.uk/medicine/story/0,,2062007,00.html).

Elgin, Tershia. *What Should I Eat? A Complete Guide to the New Food Pyramid.* New York, NY: Ballantine, 2005.

Ettlinger, Steve. *Twinkie, Deconstructed: My Journey to Discover How the Ingredients Found in Processed Foods Are Grown, Mined (Yes, Mined), and Manipulated into What America Eats.* New York, NY: Hudson Street Press, 2007.

Kesterton, Michael, quoting an article from *Harrowsmith Country Life* magazine. "Facts and Arguments," *Globe and Mail*, April 24, 2007, p. L8. ("Almost half the current Canadian herd was sired by a mere eleven bulls.")

Linn, Susan. *Consuming Kids: The Hostile Takeover of Childhood.* New York, NY: New Press, 2004.

Mittelstaedt, Martin. "'Inherently Toxic' Chemical Faces Its Future." *Globe and Mail*, Saturday, April 7, 2007, p. A10.

Nestle, Marion. *Food Politics: How the Food Industry Influences Nutrition and Health.* Berkeley, CA: University of California Press, 2003.

Nestle, Marion. *What to Eat.* New York, NY: North Point Press, 2006.

Neumark, Jill. "Autism: It's Not Just in the Head." *Discover Magazine.* April 2007, p. 33.

Pawlick, Thomas F. *The End of Food: How the Food Industry Is Destroying Our Food Supply—and What You Can Do About It.* Vancouver, BC: Greystone Books, 2006.

Pollan, Michael. *Omnivore's Dilemma: A Natural History of Four Meals.* New York, NY: Penguin, 2006.

Pollan, Michael. "You Are What You Grow." *New York Times Magazine.* NYTimes.com. April 22, 2007. Retrieved April 26, 2007 (http://www.nytimes.com/2007/04/22/magazine/22wwlnlede.t.html?...).

Schlosser, Eric. *Fast Food Nation.* New York, NY: Houghton, Mifflin, 2001.

Smith, Alisa, and J. B. MacKinnon. *The 100-Mile Diet: A Year of Local Eating.* Toronto, ON: Random House, 2007.

Spurlock, Morgan. *Don't Eat This Book: Fast Food and the Supersizing of America.* New York, NY: G. P. Putnam's Sons, 2005.

Squires, Sally. "Panel Urges Schools to Replace Junk Foods." *Washington Post,* April 25, 2007, p. A03. Retrieved June 5, 2007 (http://www.washingtonpost.com/wp-dyn/content/article/2007/04/25/AR2007042500762.html).

Index

About the Author

Paula Johanson has worked as a writer and teacher for more than twenty years. She operated an organic-method market garden for fifteen years, selling produce and sheep's wool at farmer's markets. She writes and edits nonfiction books. At two or more conferences each year, Johanson leads panel discussions on practical science and how it applies to home life and creative work. An accredited teacher, she has written and edited curriculum educational materials for the Alberta Distance Learning Centre in Canada.

Photo Credits

Cover (clockwise from top left) © Shutterstock.com, © www.istockphoto.com/creacart, © www.istockphoto.com/Rebecca Ellis, © www.istockphoto.com/Brent Shelter, © www.istockphoto.com/stocksnapper; pp. 5, 10, 28 © Jeff Greenberg/The Image Works; p. 8 © Tim Boyle/Getty Images; p. 13 © Rachel Epstein/The Image Works; p. 16 © Sarah-Maria Vischer/The Image Works; p. 19 © AP Images; p. 22 © SSPL/The Image Works; p. 26 © www.istockphoto.com/Sawayasu Tsuji; p. 31 © Voisin/Phanie/Photo Researchers, Inc.; p. 33 © www.istockphoto.com/Rohit Seth; p. 35 © Spencer Platt/Getty Images; p. 38 © www.istockphoto.com/Windzepher.

Designer: Tahara Anderson; **Editor:** Kathy Kuhtz Campbell
Photo Researcher: Amy Feinberg